# Incense

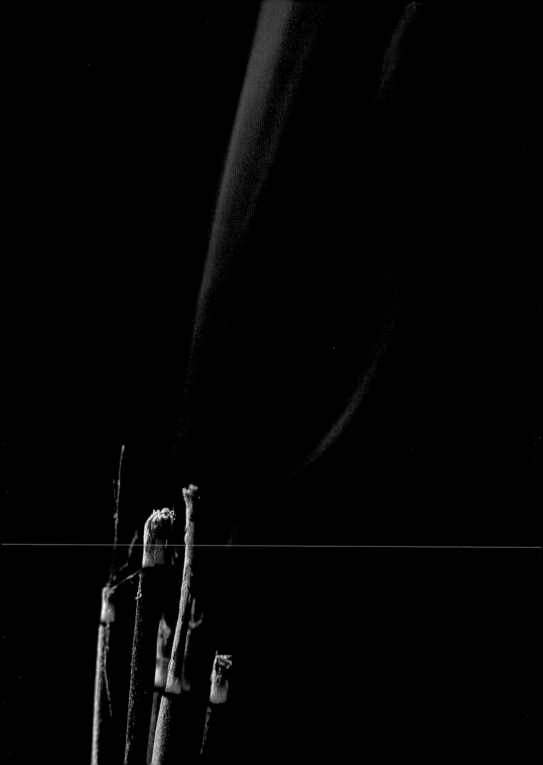

# Incense

## RITUALS ✸ MYSTERY ✸ LORE

by GINA HYAMS

Photographs by SUSIE CUSHNER

**CHRONICLE BOOKS**

SAN FRANCISCO

Text copyright © 2004 by Gina Hyams.

Photographs copyright © 1997 (pages 13, 50, and 82), 2000 (page 22), 2001 (page 47), 2002 (page 61), and 2004 by Susie Cushner.

Library of Congress Cataloging-in-Publication Data available.

ISBN 0-8118-3993-1

Manufactured in China.

Designed by Meg Coughlin
Stylist: Sara Slavin

Distributed in Canada by Raincoast Books
9050 Shaughnessy Street
Vancouver, British Columbia V6P 6E5

10 9 8 7 6 5 4 3 2 1

Chronicle Books LLC
85 Second Street
San Francisco, California 94105

www.chroniclebooks.com

For my brother,

Jan Christopher Bolling

(January 13, 1954 – January 5, 2003),

whose spirit I honor with plum wine, Rumi

and Rilke, and Tibetan incense.

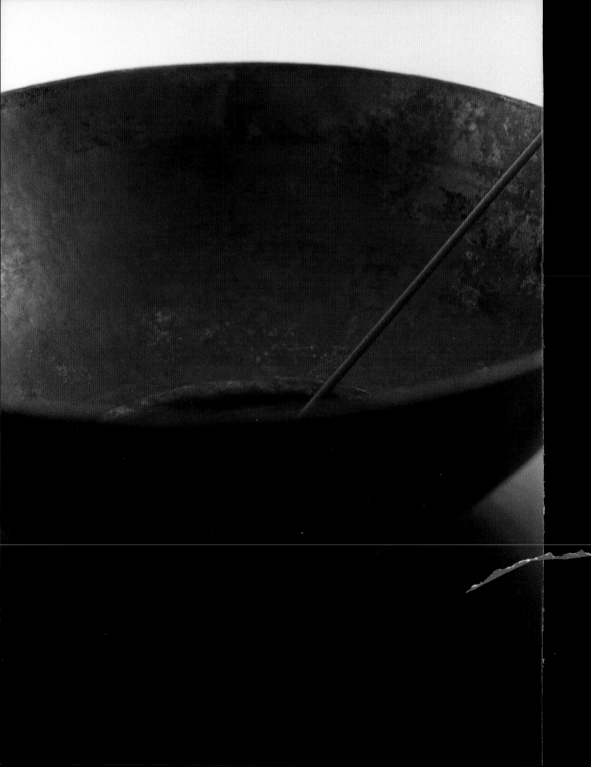

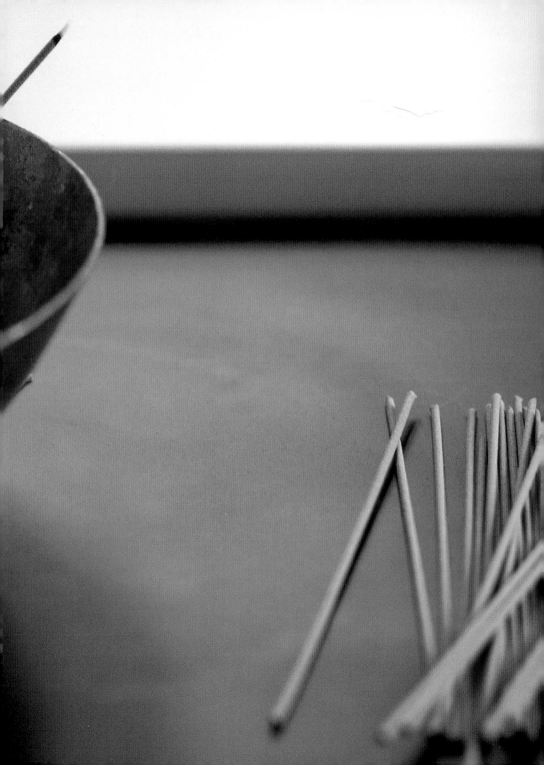

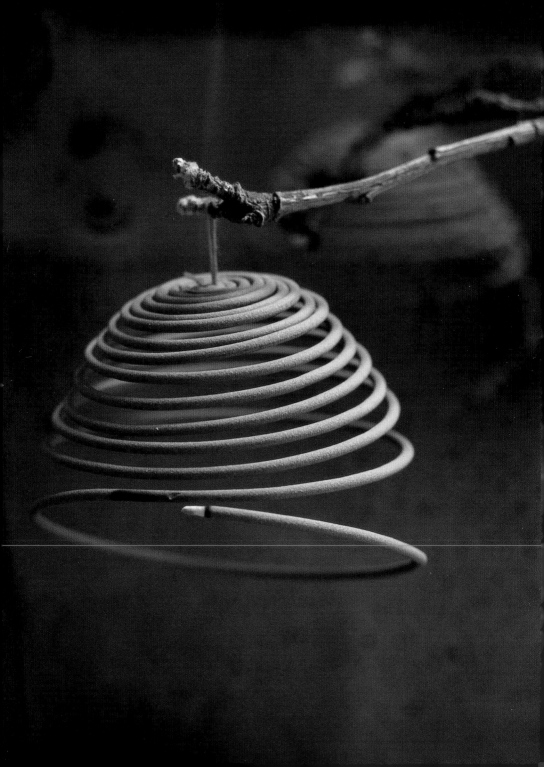

# Table of Contents

❀

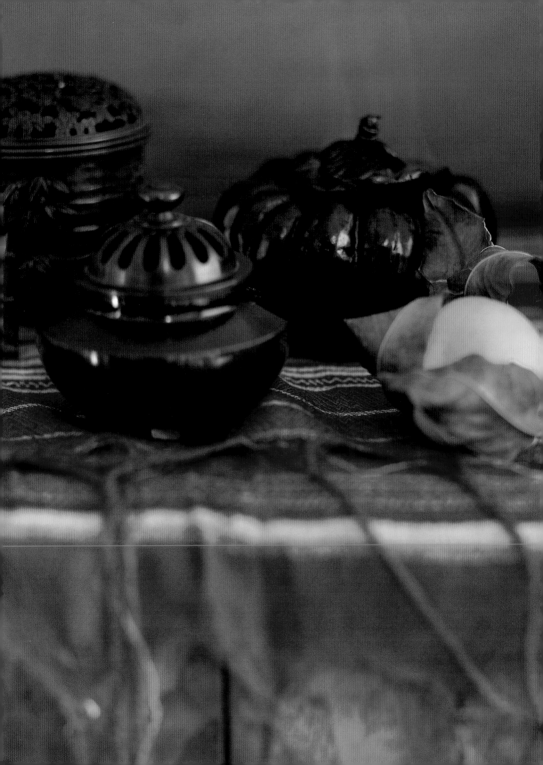

## Introduction: The Mystery of Incense

For more than five thousand years, people have burned aromatic substances in order to commune with the divine and to infuse their lives with fragrant serenity and sensual pleasure. Incense is the perfume that flowers, herbs, gums, and resins exhale when burned in celebration or as an offering to a deity. The word *incense* derives from the Latin *incensum,* which means "to set on fire." The word also means "to arouse passion or emotion."

Mandy Aftel writes in *Essence and Alchemy* that "to be immersed in a scent world, even temporarily, is to shift your consciousness and to awaken to the moment more fully." You can burn incense to help strengthen your spiritual practice, to ease your troubles in a decadent aromatic bath, to spark creativity, to promote good luck, or to kindle desire. Its sweet smoke can enhance everyday activities, such as doing chores around the house, reading books, or listening to music. Incense can be used like subtle background music, lending a mysterious air to a cocktail party or helping to banish mosquitoes at an outdoor barbecue. The heightened sense of awareness that incense inspires can also help us celebrate the major milestones in our lives—the births of children, marriage ceremonies, and memorials for loved ones.

Of the five senses, smell holds the most powerfully direct link to our emotions and memories. A single whiff of a long-forgotten fragrance can instantly provoke a cascade of memories, transporting us back through time to a precise moment and place. A whiff of juniper might trigger the memory of your first-love's cologne and the sexy, rough feel of his beard stubble when you kissed, whereas the scent of cinnamon might remind you of playing cards in your grandmother's kitchen when you were a child. The smell of pine or cedar might conjure memories of walking your dog through the woods on a crisp fall morning, the ground sparkling with dew, while the scent of frankincense might unexpectedly plunge you into melancholy, as you recall a friend's Catholic funeral.

Our reaction to smells is primal and intense because we process olfactory stimuli directly through the limbic system—the area of the brain responsible for emotion, lust, hunger, memory, and imagination. Unlike sight, sound, touch, and taste, olfactory sensation is perceived in the free-spirited right side of the brain, rather than through the analytical, rational left side. We're hardwired to feel responses to smells before we have a chance to formulate any thoughts about them.

Nearly all of the world's spiritual traditions—from Catholicism to Judaism to Buddhism to Hinduism to Islam to New Age Paganism—incorporate incense in their rituals. Incense is burned as a sacrificial offering during prayer and meditation, and while casting magic spells. During ancient times, incense was more valuable than gold, so to burn it was to sacrifice one's personal wealth for the gods. When Jesus was born, incense was so precious that, according to the authors of the

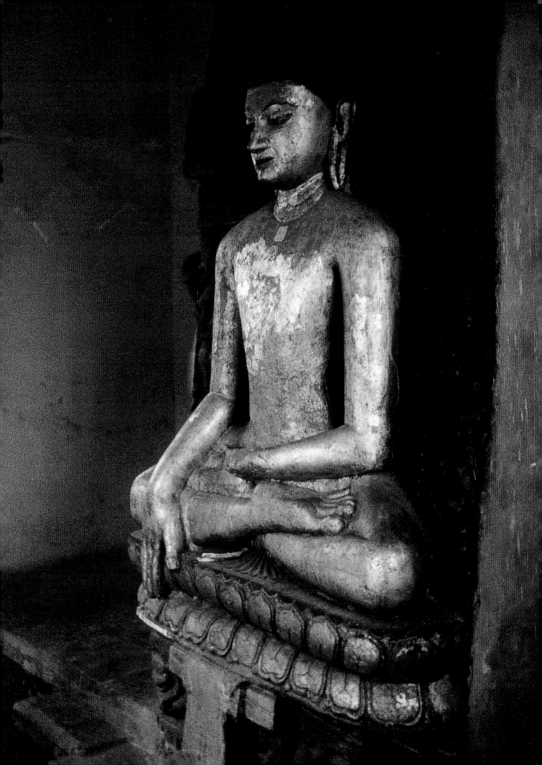

Bible, the Three Kings brought him gifts of frankincense, myrrh, and gold. Some biblical scholars speculate that the kings may have been carrying fragrant, golden-colored ambergris instead of actual gold.

Incense smoke delineates, purifies, and sanctifies sacred space. The rising clouds of fragrance carry prayers to heaven. Before modern times, incense was burned in temples and churches — places in which large groups of people gathered — also because many herbs and resins possess strong disinfectant and antiseptic properties; thus incense burning was an important sanitary measure before indoor plumbing existed.

The Japanese term for the practice of opening oneself completely to fragrance translates to "listening to incense." In the high-tech, media-saturated, conflict-ridden twenty-first century, we need the quiet truth of incense more than ever. As aromatherapist Trygve Harris explains, "Incense symbolizes and calls forth that which connects us to the ancient, to the roots and soul of the earth, to the Garden of Eden and the hand of God, to the timelessness of the spirit and the vibration of the ethereal world, to the basis of our primal selves, and the completeness of existence."

The passion for the beauty of incense and belief in its divine powers spans the globe. The ancient Egyptians (3000 B.C.–A.D. 600) were entranced with incense, burning it in sacred and medicinal rites, as well as for pleasure. Three times per day, they made offerings of incense to the sun god, Ra. At sunrise, they greeted him with smoldering resins; at noon, they ignited myrhh for him; and at sunset, they made a final offering of burning Kyphi, a magical blend of spices and herbs.

The Egyptians believed that the gods were fond of delectably sweet odors and that passage to the afterlife could be ensured if the corpse was accompanied by enough fragrance. They embalmed mummies using camphor and myrrh and lined the pharaohs' tombs with marble urns filled with aromatic spice mixtures.

Since Vedic times (1200-500 B.C.), practitioners of *Ayurvedic* holistic medicine in India have prescribed incense burning to treat physical and mental ailments. The sages of ancient India held that incense represented the idea that every human life should be like a delicate flower emitting the fragrance of good words, good deeds, and good thoughts. Even today, the air in India is still redolent with the earthy, sweet smell of sandalwood incense burned daily in religious celebrations.

In Europe, incense was an integral element of temple rites and civic celebrations. The early Greeks burned cedar, juniper, and myrrh to mask the stench of burning flesh during animal sacrifices to the gods. The priestess at Delphi inhaled smoldering sulfuric mineral and bay laurel leaf fumes to induce her prophetic trance.

The Roman emperor Nero (A.D. 100), who reportedly perfumed his palace fountains and slept on a bed of rose petals, is said to have spent the equivalent of $100,000 to scent just one party with a staggering quantity of incense. Records show that during this era Rome imported some 2,800 tons of frankincense and 550 tons of myrrh per year. The Romans, in fact, were so taken with incense that they called their loved ones "my myrrh" and "my cinnamon," in the manner that we modern-day sugar devotees use the endearments "cupcake" and "sweetie pie."

The world's voracious appetite for fragrance made rulers of the Arabian kingdom extremely wealthy during this era. Their rocky desert was the key source of frankincense, myrrh, and aloeswood. Following the twenty-four-hundred-mile-long Incense Trail, which stretched from what is now southern Oman through Yemen and Saudi Arabia to Petra, a port in Jordan, caravans of as many as three thousand camels exported the precious resins by the ton. Their journey intersected the Silk Route, thus extending incense trade to Europe and Asia.

In addition to enjoying the profits from their exports, the Arabs reveled in their region's bounty of fragrant delights. The Islamic prophet Muhammad said that the three things he loved most in this world were prayers, women, and pleasant fragrances. To this day, Yemeni women burn incense to perfume their clothing with a seductive medley of musk, aloeswood, sandalwood, clove, and rose.

The Japanese have a venerable tradition of taking the aesthetics of incense appreciation to exquisite heights. Before modern times, members of the court practiced the refined art of the Kodo incense ceremony, as well as the art of flower arranging and the tea ceremony. Men and women scented their kimonos, their rooms, and their writing paper with signature blends of incense. Up until the mid-1900s, geishas used incense clocks to track their services, billing callers according to how many incense sticks had burned during their visit. It is traditional in Japan to name especially large pieces of precious aloeswood and treat them as state treasures and family heirlooms. Some of these prized pieces of incense are more than fifteen hundred years old.

Native Americans have long infused traditional ceremonies with the pungent smoke of sage, tobacco, and sweet grass. Since pre-Hispanic times, indigenous peoples in Latin America have smoldered copal resin, believing they can see their ancestral deities in the billowing clouds of smoke. The Mayans of Mexico believe that when copal is burned, it transforms into otherworldly tortillas that the deities eat. Indigenous shamans in Latin America make extensive use of herbs and resins, interpreting omens in patterns of smoke, and determining the root of a person's fear by tossing burning copal into water — once cooled, the underside of the resin is thought to reveal a picture of what caused the fright.

Incense is a potent metaphor for the sweet, ephemeral nature of life itself. The ritual scenting of our surroundings calms the frenzy of everyday existence. It also heightens our awareness of breath and the preciousness of time. This book explores the fascinating history and lore of incense around the world, delving into the meaning of various scents and offering practical suggestions for rituals to help you incorporate the benefits of incense into your life. Consider these pages an invitation to relax and savor the earth's aromatic treasures — to kindle both body and soul as the smoke unfurls.

**The Many Forms of Incense**

*A day without fragrance is a day lost.*     ANCIENT EGYPTIAN SAYING

One Japanese manufacturer has likened incense burning to "rambling through a fantastic garden in full bloom." Each type of incense — from simple bundles of dried sage to complex Tibetan formulas containing some one hundred different ingredients, including ground semi-precious stones — can be regarded as a wonderful plant in such a garden.

There are two general types of incense: combustible and noncombustible. Combustible varieties usually contain pulverized charcoal and/or potassium nitrate (also known as saltpeter) to aid in burning, whereas the latter do not. Noncombustible incense must be smoldered on charcoal blocks or burned directly in a fire to release its fragrance. Use charcoal blocks specifically formulated for incense, since briquettes meant for outdoor grills emit toxic levels of carbon monoxide.

Some Japanese incense manufacturers utilize makko powder, a natural burning agent derived from the bark of an evergreen tree, as a healthful alternative to potassium nitrate. Some Indian companies use toxin-free charcoal made from charred coconut husks. When smoldering loose herbs and resins, you can use incense blocks derived from bamboo or glowing hot embers from wood fires instead of regular incense charcoal blocks that contain potassium nitrate.

Combustible forms of incense include joss sticks, which either have a bamboo reed down the center or are made of pure incense dough without any skewer (these sticks are solid throughout, like a piece of dried spaghetti). The thicker the bamboo, the longer the incense stick will burn, but the fragrance may be less subtle than those made of pure dough, since the smoke includes the smell of the burning skewer as well as the incense. Combustible incense dough also gets molded into cylinders, coils, spirals, and cones. The Vietnamese make enormous incense coils

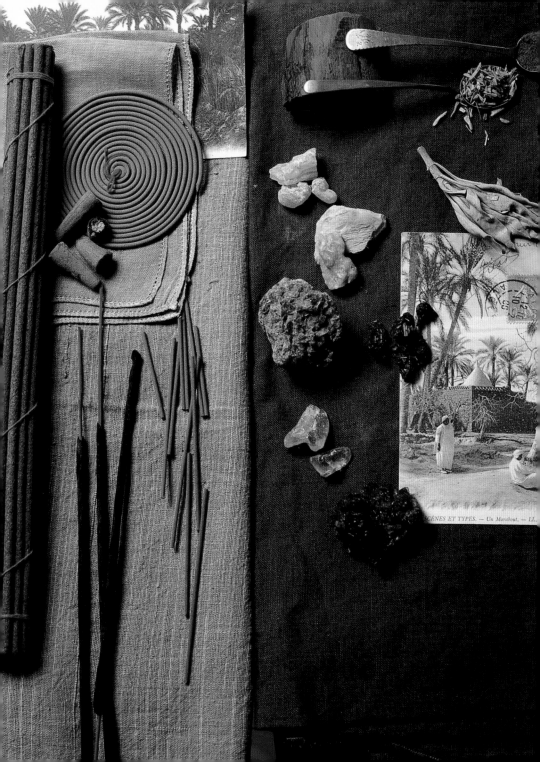

SCÈNES ET TYPES. — Un Marabout. — LL.

to hang from their temple ceilings. These coils are so large that they can burn for several days straight.

Noncombustible varieties include loose mixtures of ground dried herbs, incense pellets (dried herbs to which soft resins, balsams, dried fruits, or honey have been added), aromatic wood chips, powders, gums, and resins. Blends containing large amounts of gums and resins (frankincense and myrrh, for example) will burn longer than those composed primarily of woods and leaves.

Making incense is both an art and a science. Around the world, incense recipes and manufacturing techniques have been handed down from generation to generation in an unbroken oral tradition. Incense manufacturers fiercely guard their formulas from their competitors. The trade secrets lie in the exact proportions of ingredients and precise techniques: using the right measurements of leaves, flowers, roots, woods, resins, gums, spices, and oils; mixing them just so with the proper amount of water, wine, honey, plum paste, or sacrificial blood; rolling the dough onto sticks or molding it into particular shapes; and drying the incense in the shade or burying it underground for the perfect number of days or even years.

The best incenses are made from unadulterated, natural ingredients, free from synthetic additives and binders. The smoke from artificial ingredients can cause headaches, coughing, and eye inflammation. Cheap incense, often in cloyingly sweet flavors like strawberry, pineapple, and peach, tends to be made by dipping "punk" sticks (bamboo slivers coated in sawdust and glue) into harshly scented chemical solutions.

A strong odor, detectable through the sealed package, is one clue that an incense contains artificial ingredients. Most natural incense releases little aroma before it's heated. The strong synthetic fragrance is due to volatile chemicals oxidizing and means that the scent is only on the surface of the stick. Artificial incense produces thick, black smoke and heavy odors, unlike the smoke of natural incense, which isn't excessive and dissipates rapidly while its aroma lingers in the air.

The magic of incense lies in the belief that when natural substances burn, the power stored in the plant materials is released — the energy of earth, sunshine, rain, wind, stars, and moonlight. Each fragrance, like a color or a sound, possesses a particular vibrational quality. Synthetic oils that simulate nature may smell pleasant, but they don't contain any life force.

Incense supplies are sold by natural-foods stores, nurseries, religious and occult supply stores, incense and aromatherapy shops, and many online retailers. An economical way to experience a range of incenses is to purchase a sample pack. When you travel abroad, be sure to scour local markets for rare and exotic incenses to add to your collection.

Common incense ingredients fall into the following fragrance classifications:

*Woody:* sandalwood, cedarwood, pine, aloeswood, borneo camphor

*Spicy:* cardamom, cinnamon, clove, ginger, juniper, myrtle, basil

*Earthy:* patchouli, vetiver, oakmoss

*Balsamic:* benzoin, peru balsam, storax, tolu balsam

*Resinous:* frankincense, myrrh

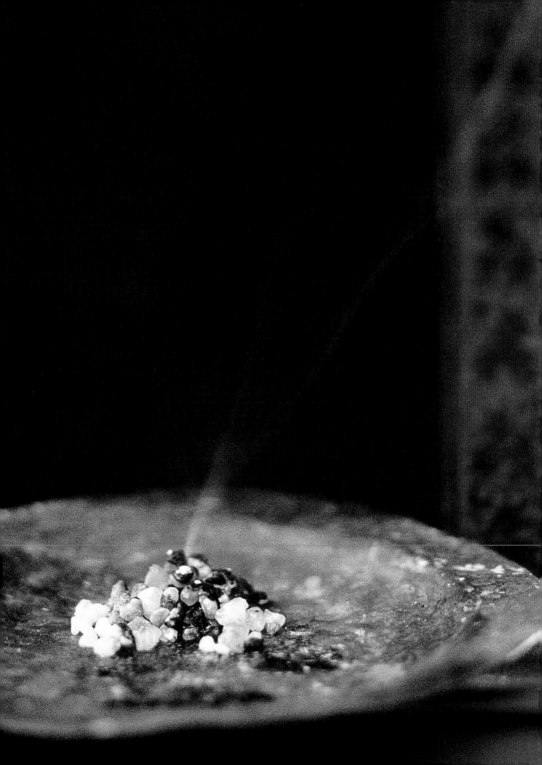

*Floral:* rose, jasmine, ylang-ylang, gardenia, honeysuckle, white lotus, orange blossom

*Herbal:* clary sage, lavender, rosemary, sweet grass

*Citrus:* citronella, lemongrass

*Animal:* musk, ambrette seeds, ambergris

Rather than classify an incense according to its horticultural or animal origin, the ancient Chinese invented six scent groups based on the sentiment evoked when the substance was burned.

Tranquility incense was enjoyed at dawn while watching the lingering moon.

Luxury incense was burned to dispel drowsiness, and Beauty incense when lovers met.

Reclusivity incense was burned in solitude to purge one's mind of earthly thoughts.

Refinement incense was burned after long hours of study to relieve mental fatigue.

Nobility incense was burned on clear, moonlit nights to keep evil spirits at bay.

Japanese incense blends are often designed to imitate aspects of nature. They are given wonderfully poetic names, such as "The Smell of the Summer Breeze," "Dew on the Mountain Path," and "Who Is There? Evening Dusk" (a scent meant to conjure the image of a lover waiting in the fading light).

Consider keeping an incense journal to note the feelings, images, memories, and lines of poetry that specific scents suggest to you. Over time, you may find that quite a few varieties become part of your own special collection that you choose from depending on your mood. On the other hand, you may discover that one fragrance fills you with such joy that it becomes your signature scent. Reactions to smells are tied to one's unique personal history and sensibility, so it's important to discover the scents that please you most. Once you find your aromatic treasures, store them in a dark, dry place to maintain their optimal scent, color, and potency.

## Incense Accessories

Incense sticks and cones should be burned in a fire-resistant ash catcher or an incense holder. You don't need to buy anything fancy to get started—just stick the incense in a bowl of sand or salt. However, should you decide to dive into the world of incense accessories, the array of elegant and whimsical designs available will astonish you.

Made of clay, stone, porcelain, jade, brass, gold, silver, seashells, and glass, incense burners can be molded to represent anything under the sun: gods and goddesses, animals, lotus blossoms, mythical dragons, log cabins with smoke coming out of the chimney, scenes of hills and mountains across which smoke wafts like mist. Noncombustible incense holders are equally diverse, ranging from the lovely raku ceramic cups used in the Japanese incense ceremony to the ornately filigreed brass censors (thuribles) employed by the Catholic Church. In Dubai, where fragrances are an integral component of daily life, automotive shops even sell electric incense burners that plug into a car's cigarette lighter. (Tip: Placing unlit incense in a hot car will freshen the air as well.)

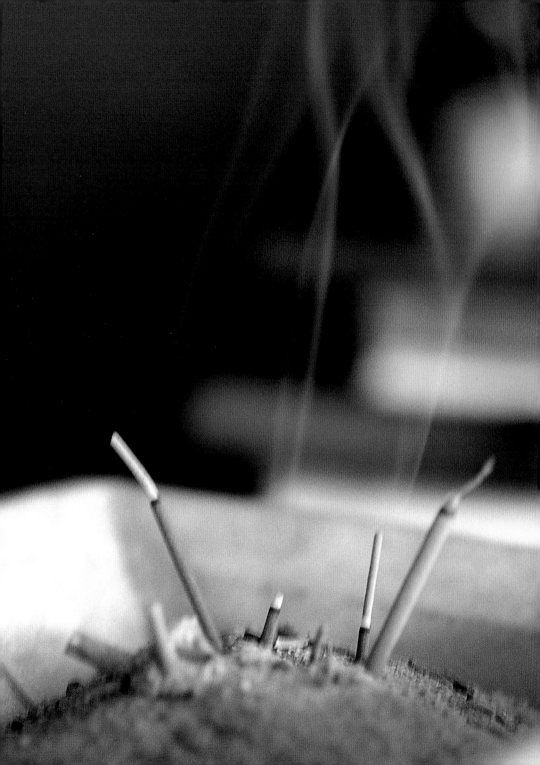

Other incense-related paraphernalia include special ash presses, feather-tipped brushes, chopsticks, spoons, tweezers, electric wood-chip heaters, mortars and pestles, storage boxes, and wafting feathers.

## How to Burn Combustible Incense

- ➤ Light the tip of the incense.

- ➤ Gently extinguish the flame by blowing or fanning, to produce a delicate wisp of smoke. (Some cultures hold that one should never blow out the flame with one's mouth because impure breath can pollute the incense.)
- ➤ For sticks, place the unlit end in the burner's holder.
- ➤ For coils and cones, gently place on the center of the burner.
- ➤ For spirals, hang from the holder.

## How to Burn Noncombustible Incense

- ➤ Fill a bowl or censer with ashes or sand.
- ➤ Hold the incense charcoal block with tweezers over a flame. If the charcoal contains potassium nitrate, tiny sparks will crackle across the surface once it is lit.
- ➤ Place the charcoal in the censer.
- ➤ When the sparks disappear, the charcoal is smoldering.
- ➤ Sprinkle a pinch or two of dried plant material or resin directly on top of or right beside the charcoal.
- ➤ When the smoke begins to thin out, add more incense.

## Incense Safety Tips

- Keep both packaged and lit incense out of the reach of children and pets.

- Secure burning incense in a nonflammable, stable holder away from drafty areas such as open windows, doors, and vents.

- Place a receptacle under the incense holder to catch falling ash.

- Never leave burning incense or charcoal unattended.

- Saturate matches, ash, and charcoal with water before discarding, since their heat can cause a fire to ignite in a wastebasket.

- If you are asthmatic, pregnant, nursing, prone to seizures, or have had a stroke, please consult a physician before using incense.

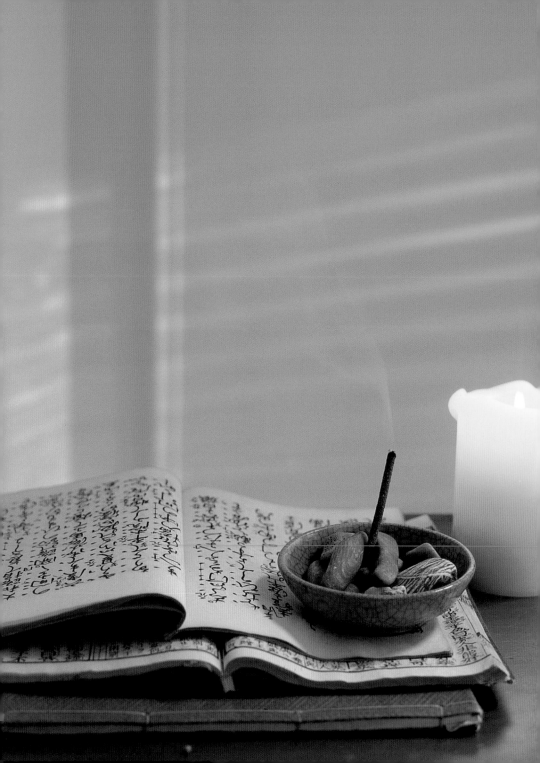

# 1 | Sacred Smoke: Incense and Spirituality

Let my prayer

be set forth before thee

as incense.

## Sacred Smoke: Incense and Spirituality

Where there is incense smoke, there is the fire of faith and prayers. Incense smoke is holy smoke. Integral to spiritual practices around the globe, its divine fragrance suffuses nearly every sort of place of worship—Hindu shrines, Catholic cathedrals, Buddhist temples, Pagan sanctuaries. When constructing mosques, Arab Muslims have gone so far as to mix musk with mortar, so that the buildings might always emit a sacred scent.

The miraculous transformation of incense from solid matter into spirit-like smoke inspires awe and reverence. Clouds of fragrance create the ambience of heaven and give a visceral sense of mystical transcendence. The consuming fire of incense, which starts at one end and doesn't stop until it reaches the other, also symbolizes religious zeal and commitment to stay the course toward enlightenment.

Throughout the world, incense is what links the earth to the spiritual realm. Different cultures view it respectively as a door, a window, a ladder, or a telephone between worlds. Worshipers in many faiths make sacrificial offerings of incense believing that its sacred smoke will transport their gratitude and prayers to the gods and goddesses, saints, or ancestral souls. For instance, according to the Bible, when

Noah arrived on dry land after surviving the flood, he thanked God by burning myrrh and cedar. When Taiwanese people are in trouble, they sometimes make offerings of "emergency incense," lighting both ends of a joss stick to signal that their prayer needs urgent attention.

According to Buddhist and Hindu lore, one should burn incense for the benefit of deities, and for the welfare and pleasure of all beings; incense represents the belief that one's actions should give happiness to others, just as herbs give away their lovely fragrance. Buddhists and Hindus believe that as the incense smoke permeates the temple, it spreads the virtues of wisdom and compassion, purifying the space and expunging evil from the hearts of those present.

### Incense for Prayer and Meditation

The fragrances that follow are traditionally burned during prayer and meditation. These aromas are known for their propensity to induce deep breathing and draw the mind toward clarity. As you develop your own spiritual rituals, experiment with these and other scents to discover which ones generate feelings of peace and communion within you. Whatever your religious beliefs, incense can serve as a bridge to the divine, bringing depth and immediacy to your prayer, meditation, yoga, or other spiritual practice.

- The haunting, rich scent of **aloeswood resin** (also known as agarswood, oud, eagle wood, jinko, and kyara) is cherished for its power to calm and center the spirit during meditation. The highest grade of aloeswood costs as much as $1,000 per gram (about a half teaspoon).

- The mild scent of **Borneo camphor** is refreshing and thought to help maintain concentration.

- The smoky, sweet fragrance of **cedarwood** is believed to promote feelings of safety and security and to inspire the virtues of integrity and fortitude.

- **Clove** smells fresh and spicy. The energizing fragrance is said to promote festive feelings and creativity.

- The rich, herbal scent of **dragon's blood** resin is believed to purify and protect.

- **Frankincense** is the gum resin of Boswellia trees. Its soothing, resinous scent is thought to elevate the mind and expand spiritual consciousness.

- The rich, spicy smell of **myrrh** resin is considered to be profoundly calming and restorative.

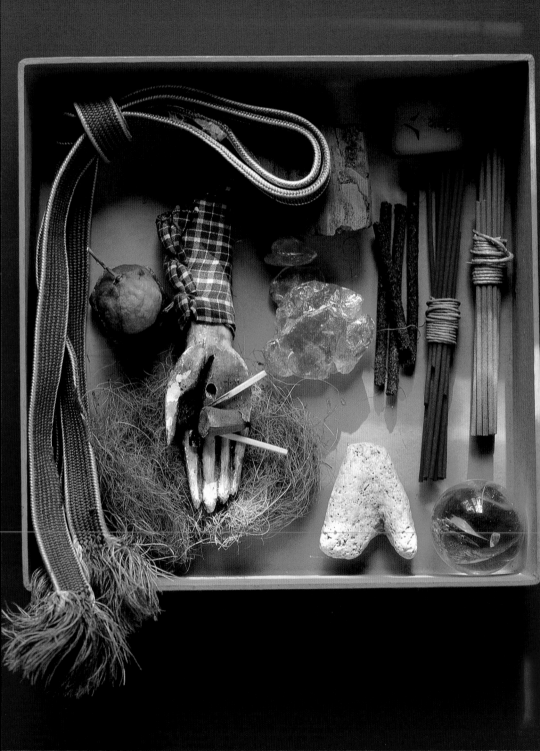

## Creating a Personal Scented Sanctuary

Focus your spiritual energies by creating a personal altar on which to burn incense. If your house is large enough to accommodate a private meditation room or chapel, that's wonderful, but the surroundings of your altar need not be grand to be effective. Your sacred space will come alive if you imbue it with your faith and commitment to living a spiritually authentic existence. You can dedicate a corner of a bedroom as your special spot for contemplation, or you can place your altar on top of a dresser, on a fireplace mantel, on a windowsill, or in a sheltered spot in your garden. Grace your incense altar with things that represent the divine for you, be they images of deities, candles, flowers, leaves, seashells, rocks, or a tabletop water fountain.

## Purifying Sacred Space

Native Americans traditionally call on the spirits of sacred plants to cleanse people and places of harmful energies, thoughts, and influences. This purification ritual, called smudging, is said to clear the atmosphere of negative vibrations caused by anger, sadness, or illness and to fill the environment with positive, uplifting feelings.

The pungent smoke of desert sage is believed to drive away negativity. Sweet grass, which smells like fresh-cut hay, is thought to attract positive energies and restore balance after a space has been cleared of negativity. The dried plants are bundled into wands called smudge sticks. Other herbs typically used in the smudging ceremony include white sage, cedar, pine, lavender, copal, mugwort, and yerba santa.

## How to Smudge a Room

- Light the bundle of herbs on fire, then blow out the flame and place the smoldering wand in a ceramic bowl or abalone shell.

- Starting in the east and moving clockwise, use a feather or your hand to gently fan the smoke into the four corners of the room as an offering to the sacred Four Directions.

- Fan the smoke so that it wafts down toward the floor to thank the Earth and up toward the ceiling to thank the Sky.

- Walk around the perimeter of the room, imagining all negativity attaching to the smoke and vanishing as it dissipates. As you do this, pray to the Great Spirit to bring peace to the room and all the people who occupy it.

- After smudging, extinguish the embers by burying the lit end of the wand in a bowl of sand.

## Three Incense Prayers

### Taoist Incense Prayer

*As the scented cinder smolders into flame,*

*So too the faith from which the Tao came.*

*As the winding wisp ascends into the sky*

*The wafting scent of heaven stirs my mind.*

*To the Superior Spirits, I respectfully pray:*

*May this gesture sway their Eminence to stay*

*If but a moment, should they deign to pass this way.*

*And at this time, as a disciple, I entreat*

*The Sky above and Earth beneath my feet.*

*May my heart immersed in hope be recognized*

*As that pure space of spirit highly prized.*

*May blessings rain on us a shower of love*

*As they make their calm descent from up above.*

### Zen Buddhist Incense Offering

Face a shrine, scroll, or Buddha image with incense, a candle, and a bell placed before it.

Place your palms together in front of your chest. This gesture, called *gassho,* is a sign of reverence and symbolizes the unity of oneself, Buddha, and the world.

Ring the bell three times, then bow.

Light the candle and recite:

> *Mindful of the Buddha of Eternal Life and Light,*
> *I calmly light this candle*
> *Brightening the face of the earth.*

Bow and ring the bell once.

Light the incense and recite:

> *In gratitude and joy, I offer this incense*
> *To Buddha of Eternal Life and Light,*
> *The teacher of gods and humans,*
> *The sovereign of all worlds.*
> *May the fragrance of this incense*
> *Help manifest in my heart and mind*
> *The fruit of understanding.*

Bow and ring the bell once.

Recite:

> *I take refuge in Buddha.*
> *I take refuge in the Dharma.*
> *I take refuge in Sangha.*

Bow three times.

**Zuni Incense Prayer**

*Beseeching the breath of the divine one,*

*His life-giving breath,*

*His breath of old age,*

*His breath of waters,*

*His breath of seeds,*

*His breath of riches,*

*His breath of fecundity,*

*His breath of power,*

*His breath of strong spirit,*

*His breath of all good fortune whatsoever,*

*Asking for his breath*

*And into my warm body drawing his breath,*

*I add to your breath*

*That happily you may always live.*

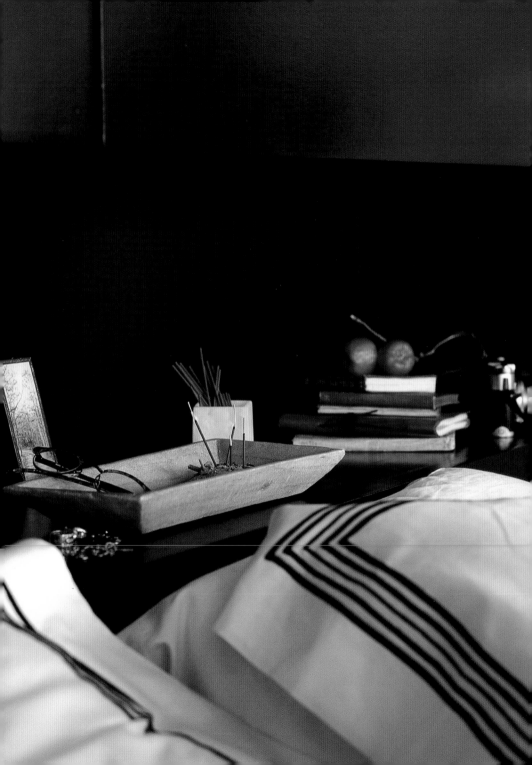

# 2 | Kindling Desire: Incense and Romance

I have perfumed my bed

    With myrrh, aloes, and cinnamon.

Come, let us take our fill of love

        until morning;

    Let us delight ourselves with love.

PROVERBS 7:17-18

## Kindling Desire: Incense and Romance

The ancient Egyptian queen Cleopatra well understood the power of fragrance to ignite desire. Preparing to seduce Marc Antony, she ordered attendants to perfume everything around her. The sails of her barge were drenched with henna blossoms and jasmine; her bedroom floor strewn knee-deep with rose petals; and her skin and clothing infused with the smoke of winter's bark, sandalwood, orris root, patchouli, myrrh, and frankincense. Dazzled by the fragrant splendor, Marc Antony had no choice but to surrender to Cleopatra's allure. As Shakespeare described it, even "the winds were love-sick."

Aromas have the glorious ability to subvert the rational mind. A whiff of luscious incense carries us instantly from the high-pressure world of endless to-do lists to the realm of carnal mystery. The delicious smoke clears our minds and returns us to our bodies. It stirs primal energies, readying our bodies to touch and be touched. The ritual burning of incense is a way to nurture and cultivate our sensual selves. It's why so many love songs contain the rhyming words "fire" and "desire." Smoldering incense in the bedroom is an invitation to burn with passion.

The classic Indian text *Kama Sutra,* written more than three thousand years ago, celebrates sex as a pathway to spiritual bliss. The book describes aromatics as being key to the art of love. The environment most conducive to facilitating divine union was thought by the author to be a pungent bedroom, thick with the smell of jasmine garlands, sandalwood incense, and the sweat of ecstasy.

Just as the alluring aroma of flowers attracts bees, butterflies, and other pollinating creatures, floral fragrances function as aphrodisiacs in the human kingdom as well. Diane Ackerman writes in *A Natural History of the Senses* that the essence of flowers "reminds us in vestigial ways of fertility, vigor, life force, all the optimism, expectancy, and passionate bloom of youth. We inhale its ardent aroma and, no matter what our ages, we feel young and nubile in a world aflame with desire."

Earthy, spicy scents such as cinnamon, ginger, nutmeg, and clove have long been known for their aphrodisiac properties. A study by the Smell and Taste Research Foundation supported this folk wisdom with the scientific finding that pumpkin pie mixed with lavender is the odor men find most sexually arousing.

Consider spicing up your bedroom with the romantic incense aromas described below.

- ➤ The warm, spicy smell of **cinnamon** is thought to be emotionally uplifting and restorative.
- ➤ **Clary sage** is said to help overcome inhibitions and banish feelings of grief. It has a nutty, herbaceous odor.
- ➤ The fiery sweetness of **ginger**'s fragrance is said to be revitalizing.

- Hindu poets call **jasmine** "Moonlight of the Grove." Its sweet, seductive scent is believed to restore balance and confidence, and to encourage feelings of optimism and openness.

- Sensual, rich, and gamy, **musk** derives from the scent gland of the musk deer. Unfortunately, due to the popularity of this aphrodisiac, the animal is now an endangered species. Herbal substitutes for musk include ambrette seeds, spikenard roots, and musk thistle flowers.

- Tender and sweet, **rose** symbolizes love and compassion. Its reassuring fragrance is believed to produce feelings of joyful well-being.

- The invigorating, herbal scent of **rosemary** is believed to dispel confusion and to inspire fidelity.

- The creamy, sweet scent of **ylang-ylang** is thought to help overcome barriers to intimacy such as nervousness, anger, and frigidity. The delicate yellow flowers are placed on wedding beds in Indonesia.

Explore a range of incenses to discover which ones move you and your lover. The nineteenth-century French emperor Napoleon Bonaparte is said to have been partial to rosemary, whereas his wife, Josephine, preferred the aroma of musk. The walls and draperies of Josephine's bedroom are said to still exude the lingering fragrance of the musk she relished so often. When Napoleon was away in battle, he burned incense before his wife's portrait so that he might feel as if she were nearby.

The power of incense to create a romantic atmosphere is vividly evoked in the ancient Japanese love story, *The Tale of Genji*, by Lady Murasaki Shikibu. Written circa A.D. 1025, the novel provides a glimpse into the lives of the Japanese aristocrats of the time. Members of the court played sophisticated incense games and created their own signature blends of incense to scent their clothing and living quarters. Shikibu describes the palace at night:

> "Under the wonderful glow of a slightly clouded moon,
>
> The rain just stopped—the wind moved gently,
>
> Dispersing the beautiful fragrance of flowers.
>
> Throughout the palace, this fragrance was joined by
>
> The unbelievably delicate fragrance of incense burning
>
> Creating a mood of enchantment."

Infusing bedroom air with the languorous drama of incense signals that the time spent there is truly a special event. Turn off the television. Dim the lights. Breathe deeply. Allow your heart to relax, open, and soften. Let your body burn along with the incense. Feast and luxuriate in the smoke.

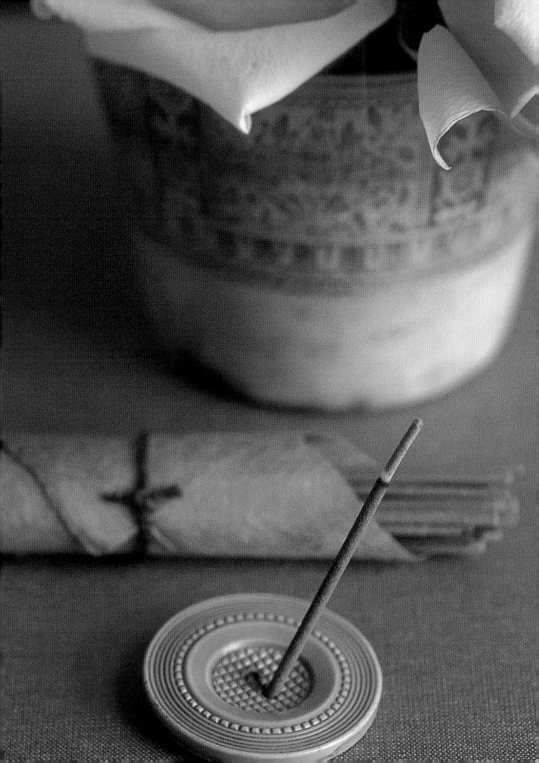

## Scenting the Body and Clothing

Veiled women in the Muslim world scent their *burkas* and *chadors* with bakhur, a chunky rose-water-and-sugar-based incense. Each family concocts their own unique recipe, but most contain cardamom, musk, amber, aloeswood, essential oils, and ground conch shells known as *duffer*. These ingredients are blended in a big pot and cooked with sugar, which is used as a binder. When placed on a bit of charcoal, the incense smokes and bubbles, releasing a tremendously sweet, rich aroma that clings to clothing, skin, and hair. In Yemen today, women are covered from head to toe (all you see is their eyes) but the fragrant cloud that follows them is one of the most alluring and sensual things in the world.

To scent your body, when you step out of the bath, slather your skin with oil and then stand over a smoking incense censor. The smoke will perfume your damp skin and hair.

## Other Romantic Suggestions

### INCENSE SACHETS

Scent your lingerie and linens with handmade incense sachets. Sachets make wonderful gifts and are easy to sew. Search boutique fabric stores for unusual remnants and check antique shops for vintage embroidered handkerchiefs and cocktail napkins that can make beautiful, instantly decorated little pouches. Pieces of worn-out kimonos, old silk night-gowns, hand-loomed ikat fabric, and patterned felt are other fun choices. Fill your sachets with broken bits of incense, pulverized woods and spices, or dried flower petals and herbs. Classic sachet mixtures include dried lavender and rose blossoms; ground sandalwood, oakmoss, and orris root; and dried rosemary, mint leaves, thyme, and ground cloves.

*Directions*

Cut out two pieces of fabric in the size you'd like, for example, 4 inches by 4 inches, or 2 inches by 5 inches; add 1/4 inch to each edge for a seam. Place the front sides together and stitch along three sides of the rectangle or square, leaving one end open. Turn the pouch inside out, then decorate the cover with a combination of ribbons, lace, buttons, beads, feathers, embroidery, and silk flowers. Fill the pouch one-half to three-quarters full with incense or potpourri. Either cinch the top closed with a ribbon or fold the fabric down toward the inside and sew it shut. Keep your stitches small; if they get too large, the stuffing will leak out.

If you prefer, purchase ready-made sachet pouches at a craft-supply shop and fill them with premixed potpourri, or simply store sticks of unlit incense amid your silk nothings and satin sheets.

FRAGRANT LOVE LETTERS

Burn your favorite incense while composing a love letter. The smoke will delicately scent the paper and give the recipient an aromatic reminder of you when he or she opens the envelope. For a more intense fragrance, dust your stationery with a sprinkling of ground incense or dried flower petals and herbs. You can even scent your ink by adding two to six drops of essential oil per teaspoon of ink. Consider writing with patchouli-scented

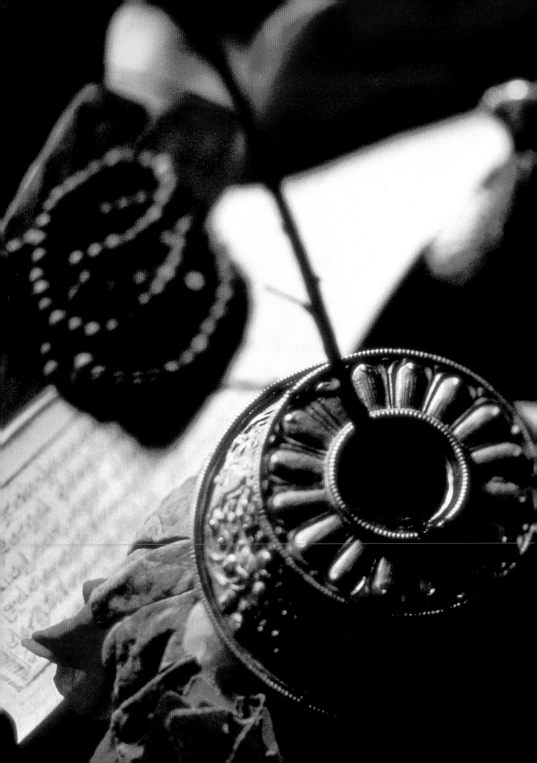

rich brown ink on clove-dusted parchment, or with jasmine-perfumed emerald green ink on handmade rose-petal paper. If you are writing to your beloved after an argument, you might smudge the paper by burning sage and sweet grass to help dispel the tension between you. Whatever fragrance you choose, be sure to seal your missive with a kiss.

## CAST A LOVE SPELL

According to Pagan witchcraft tradition, the first Friday after a new moon is the best time to cast love spells. To construct your love altar, drape a small table with a lush red fabric — something luxurious like crimson silk, ruby-colored velvet, or scarlet satin. Place a stick of sweet-smelling rose incense and two candles at the center of the table. Use red candles to draw passionate romance or pink candles for affectionate friendship. Adorn the altar with tokens that symbolize love to you, such as a long-stemmed rose, a pair of champagne flutes, a Shakespeare sonnet, or a photo of the one you desire. Light the candles and the incense. Look into the burning ember tip of the incense and recite aloud the spell below. According to Witch Bree, author of *Witch's Brew: Good Spells for Love,* it will create loving magic.

> *Venus, cast your light on me,*
> *A Goddess for today I'll be.*
> *A lover, strong and brave and true,*
> *I seek as a reflection of you.*

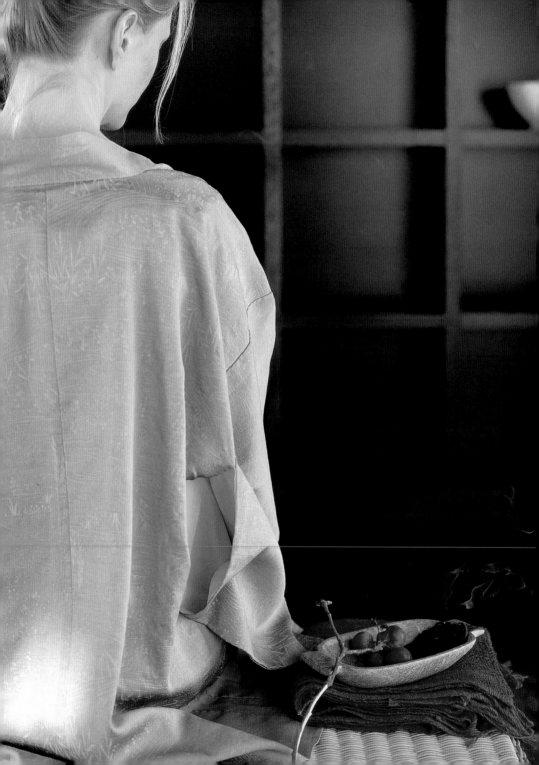

# 3 Living in Harmony: Incense and Well-Being

Look at the perfume of flowers

And of nature for peace of mind

And joy in life

Wang Wei (Chinese poet, eighth century a.d.)

# Living in Harmony: Incense and Well-Being

For thousands of years, incense has played a central role in the tradi- tional healing practices of India, Tibet, and China. The essential oils contained in incense are believed to cure a vast array of mental and physical ailments — everything from headaches and indigestion to insomnia and psychosis.

*Ayurveda* (the Science of Life) is an ancient holistic medical system based on Indian Hindu philosophy. Its premise is that all diseases are caused by some imbalance in a person's inner life. People get sick when they forget the rules of living in harmony with nature. They experience unhealthy feelings, such as hate, jealousy, greed, selfishness, and vanity. One of the first physical manifestations of such an imbalance is an irregular breathing pattern.

Ayurvedic practitioners examine a patient's physical constitution, current emotional state, stage of life, and social order. Once the doctor determines a diagnosis, he or she then considers the intrinsic qualities of flowers and herbs to select a precise single or compound aromatic to bring harmony to the individual. The incense helps patients to reestab-lish a deep, rhythmic breathing pattern and, in the process, to begin to heal and gain perspective on their condition. Daily use of incense is thought to purify the air, remove negative influences, and increase *prana* (life force).

Hindus believe that the five aspects of existence – earth, air, fire, water, and space – are divinely interconnected and that anguish-filled feelings of duality and separateness are caused by ignorance. Incense cultivates a sense of balance and interconnection because its smoke gently permeates both the external physical environment and the internal space of one's body, thus eliminating duality. To breathe in incense smoke is to breathe in nature's wisdom.

Hippocrates, considered the father of Western medicine, also believed in the healing power of scent. Circa 400 B.C., the Greek physician proclaimed that "the best way to health is to have an aromatic bath and a scented massage every day." Indeed, incense could be called the original aromatherapy product, embraced for its healing properties long before such things as scented candles and essential-oil atomizing rings existed.

Reflecting on the effect of using fragrance in her beauty routine, Japanese courtesan Lady Shonegon (circa A.D. 1000) noted in her diary that "to wash one's hair, make one's toilette, and put on scented robes – even if not a soul sees one, these preparations still produce an inner pleasure." More than offering superficial pampering, natural scents fortify our spirits.

To enjoy incense, you've got to take time to stop and smell the roses – or the sandalwood, as the case may be. There is simply no point in rushing it. For this reason, in addition to the many relaxing benefits of fragrance,

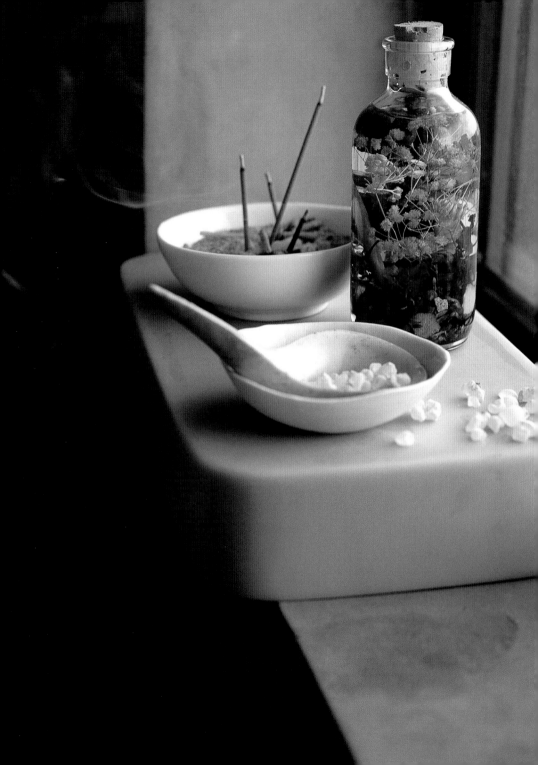

burning incense is a great way to unwind after a busy day. As a stick of incense transforms from brown paste into sweet smoke, so too can you transform yourself into the calm, creative, and loving person you want to be.

You can also use incense to set a harmonious mood when you entertain friends and family. As guests enter your party, they'll be enveloped by the gently spiced air and instantly feel at ease. At outdoor gatherings, incense smoke can help banish mosquitoes and other pests. Citronella, copal, and lavender are effective insect repellents. Always be mindful of fire hazard and use adequate-size holders and censers, so that the burning embers are protected from the wind.

Loose incense mixtures and incense pellets can be thrown directly into outdoor campfires or indoor fireplaces. Incense smolders best on glowing coals rather than in direct flame, though, so either wait until the fire dies down or create suitable coals by placing a few stones around the outer rim of the fire and sprinkle the incense on them when they become sufficiently hot. Alternatively, use tongs to place coals from the fire into a heat-resistant container, such as a ceramic flower pot, and then sprinkle the incense on top.

The following incense fragrances are known for their soothing and uplifting properties.

- Fresh and spicy, **basil** is thought to improve concentration and strengthen feelings of empathy.
- The rich, vanilla-like scent of **benzoin** resin is believed to be comforting.

- The smoky, sweet smell of **juniper** is said to be emotionally restorative.

- Sweet and mellow, **lavender** is said to have a steadying influence on the psyche, helping to temper mood swings and relieve insomnia.

- The light, refreshing fragrance of **myrtle** is thought to heal old emotional wounds and to promote forgiveness.

- The sensual, herbaceous scent of **patchouli** is believed to help put problems into perspective and to increase feelings of joy.

- **Storax** produces a grassy, sweet smell that is said to ease insomnia.

## Morning Calm Ritual

To begin your day with peaceful clarity, place a mini stick of Japanese incense in a holder and a lighter on your nightstand before you fall asleep. Set your alarm clock for ten minutes earlier than the time you really need to get out of bed. If you have a clock radio, tune it to a jazz or classical music station and set the volume low.

When your alarm sounds in the morning, roll over and hit the snooze button, or let the tranquil music play. Wiggle your fingers and toes and stretch like a cat. Gradually ease your body up to a seated position, and then slowly open your eyes. As you light the incense, admire the flickering dance of the flame and feel its warmth before blowing it out with a deep exhalation. Breathe in. Let the mellow fragrance coax your consciousness from night into day, from the realm of dreams to that of work and play. Even this brief interlude of serenity first thing upon waking can help you feel settled and strong, prepared to face any challenges ahead.

## Big Sky Meditation

When you're feeling overwhelmed or burdened by petty yet all-consuming daily concerns like office politics or computer crashes, taking incense out-of-doors can help you gain a healthy, holistic perspective. Glass bottle incense holders are ideal for outdoor incense burning because the ash settles at the bottom of the bottle, where it's sheltered from the wind. The clever design reduces fire hazard and simplifies incense transportation and cleanup.

Settle yourself comfortably before a sweeping vista. Depending on where you live, you might choose to sit on a bluff overlooking the sea, at a lookout on the rim of a verdant canyon, or on the rooftop of your urban apartment building. Secure a stick of incense in the ring or cork stopper that came with your incense bottle. Light the incense and blow out the flame, then place the smoldering end of the stick into the bottle through the side hole until the stopper holds it in place. An ethereal tendril of smoke will rise up like a genie from the bottle's spout.

As you gaze into the vast horizon, breathe deeply, and feel the day-to-day clutter in your mind fall away. Draw inspiration from the wonder of the sky—its profound blue, the billowing clouds, or its sparkling constellation of midnight stars. Breathe into the big picture. Imagine the space within your body as continuous with the space outside. Find solace in the unobstructed view. A feeling of wholeness will follow.

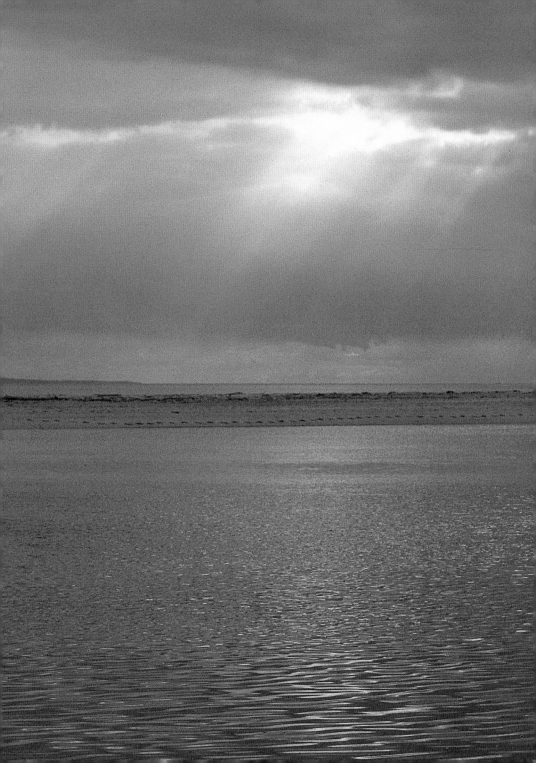

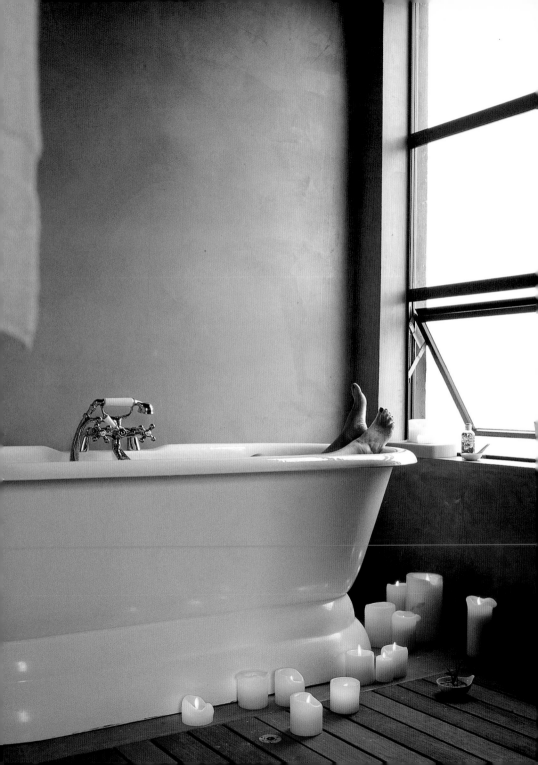

## Bubbles and Smoke

For the ultimate sensory immersion, infuse your bathwater with scent by using essential oils or bubble bath, and imbue the air with a complementary scent of incense. Light the incense while the tub is filling, so the smoke and steam fuse to create a decadent, sensual atmosphere. Surround your bathtub with votive or other candles. Toss in a handful of flower petals if you like. Submerged in the warm water, feel your breath moving in and out of your body like an ocean wave. With every exhalation, imagine your anxieties drifting away and vanishing with the smoke.

## Three Incense Baths

| CALMING BATH | REFRESHING BATH | SENSUAL BATH |
| --- | --- | --- |
| Burn frankincense incense. | Burn cinnamon incense. | Burn sandalwood incense. |
| Add to the bathwater: | Add to the bathwater: | Add to the bathwater: |
| 6 drops of lavender oil | 4 drops of neroli oil | 3 drops of jasmine oil |
| | 2 drops of ylang-ylang oil | 3 drops of rose oil |

## Sweet Dreams, Egyptian Style

The most sacred of the ancient Egyptian incenses was called Kyphi (which translates as "Welcome to the Gods"). High priests concocted Kyphi during secret, chant-filled temple ceremonies. The incense was said to consist of "things that delight in the night." Greek historian Plutarch (A.D. 46-120) wrote that smelling Kyphi was like "listening to beautiful music." He also described it as having the power to "rock a person to sleep, brighten dreams, and chase away the troubles of the day."

A great many recipes for making Kyphi exist. The following is an intoxicating yet easy-to-make version.

## KYPHI INCENSE

| | |
|---|---|
| 4 raisins | 1/2 teaspoon frankincense |
| 1 tablespoon red wine | 1/2 teaspoon benzoin |
| 1 teaspoon sandalwood | 1/4 teaspoon myrrh |
| 1/4 teaspoon juniper berries | 1/4 teaspoon dragon's blood |
| 1/4 teaspoon orris root | 1/2 teaspoon honey |
| 1/4 teaspoon cinnamon | |

Soak the raisins in the red wine overnight.

Using a mortar and pestle, individually grind the sandalwood, juniper berries, orris root, and cinnamon. In a large wooden or ceramic bowl, mix the dry ingredients together.

Using a mortar and pestle, individually pulverize the frankincense, benzoin, myrrh, and dragon's blood into small granules. Add the resins and gums to the powder mixture.

Drain the red wine from the raisins and mash the raisins with the mortar and pestle. Add the raisins and honey to the dough. Knead thoroughly with your hands, then form the dough into pea-sized balls. Spread the balls out on wax paper and store them indoors away from direct sunlight and moisture. To facilitate even drying, turn the balls daily for one to two weeks, depending on the climate. Once they are dry, store your Kyphi balls in a sealed plastic bag or glass jar. Smolder the incense balls one or two at a time over charcoal.

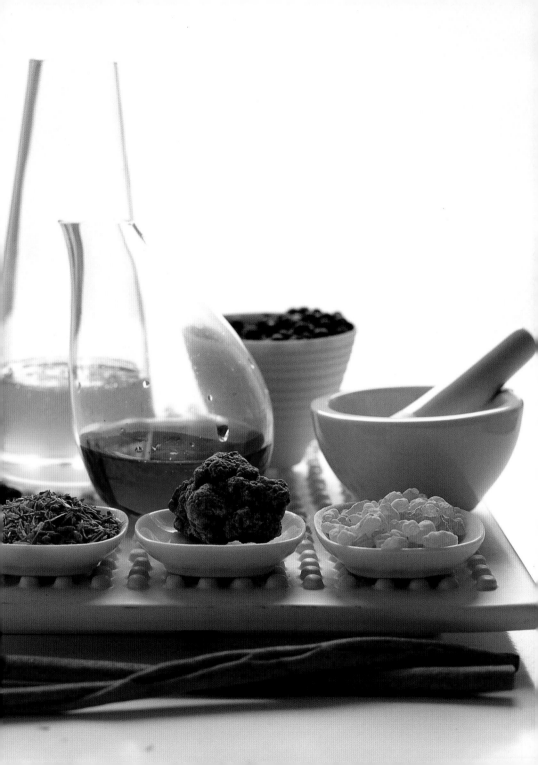

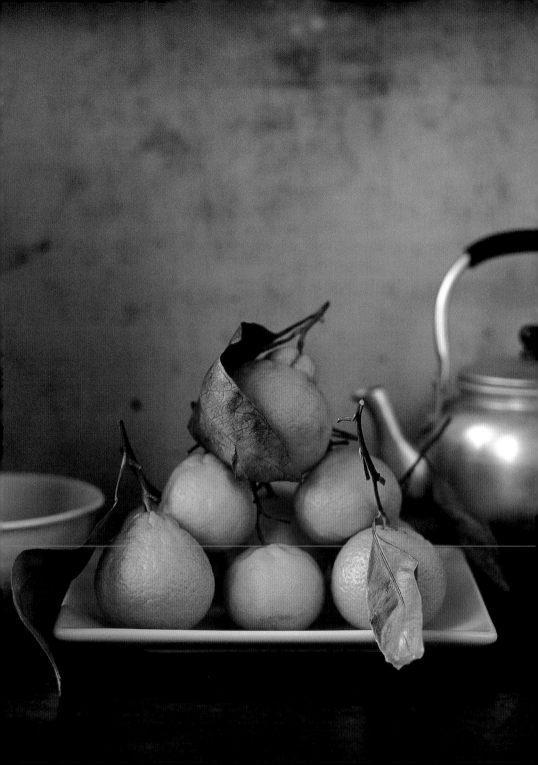

# 4 Courting the Muse: Incense and Inspiration

I don't feel like writing a poem,

Instead, I will light the incense-burning vessel

Filled with myrrh,

       jasmine,

             and frankincense,

And the poem will grow in my heart

Like the flowers in my garden.

HAFIZ (PERSIAN POET, FOURTEENTH CENTURY A.D.)

## Courting the Muse: Incense and Inspiration

Writers, musicians, and artists throughout the world have used incense as a creative tool. The magical smoke encourages flights of imagination—no surprise, considering that the word *inspiration* means "to breathe in."

For centuries, Chinese calligraphers have been partial to sandalwood for its power to calm the mind and to steady the hand, allowing creativity to flow. Balinese gamelan dancers sometimes perform wearing headdresses studded with wafting incense. The ancient Egyptians believed that benzoin stimulated creativity, and the Minoans thought anise supported intellectual endeavors. Rock musician George Harrison and sitar player Ravi Shankar used to burn durbar agarbathi Indian stick incense during their concerts.

Moved by the aroma of a madeleine (a small, light, shell-shaped cake) soaked in lime blossom tea, French writer Marcel Proust was inspired to write *Remembrance of Things Past.* In the novel, he describes the delicate yet tenacious grip that smell and taste can have on our memories: "When from a long-distant past nothing subsists, after the people are dead, after the things are broken and scattered, taste and smell alone, more fragile but more enduring, more unsubstantial, more

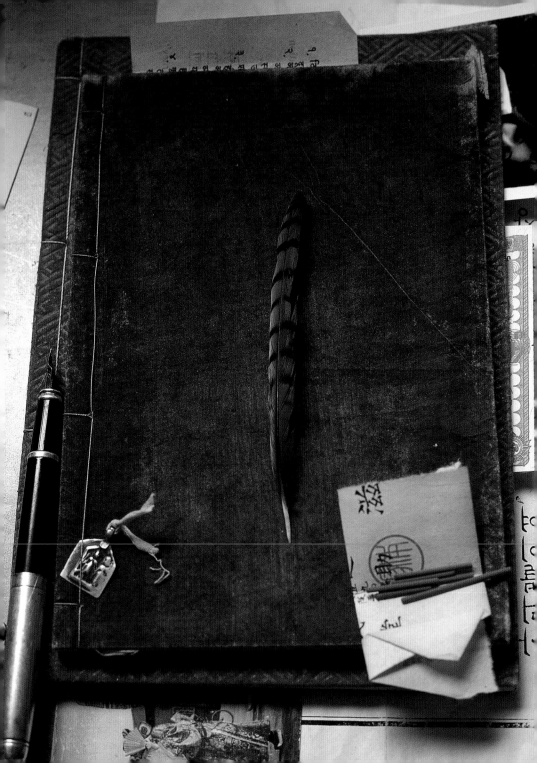

persistent, more faithful, remain poised a long time, like souls, remembering, waiting, hoping, amid the ruins of all the rest; and bear unflinchingly, in the tiny and almost impalpable drop of their essence, the vast structure of recollection."

You too can use scent to mine your memory as inspiration for your artistic pursuits. Incorporate incense into your own creative practice — be it a formal art form, knitting, or dancing your heart out in your living room.

### Incense and Journal Writing

When you sit down to write in your journal, light incense to deepen both your breath and your thoughts. The fragrant smoke will help turn your attention inward. First take three slow breaths, then begin each journal entry by describing how your body feels in that particular moment, to ground yourself fully in the present. Where are you holding tension? What is that knot in your right shoulder about? Why does your stomach feel fluttery with butterflies? Follow the aroma of the incense as it flows through your body and suffuses your thoughts. Let your words flow with equal ease. Don't worry about punctuation or spelling. If you pay close attention to your thoughts and feelings, your words will be vivid and authentic, leading you to make surprising discoveries about yourself.

## Japanese-Inspired Incense Games

*"If one can suspend any preconceptions about incense to fully experience the ceremony, the happy result will be the ability to appreciate 'incense time' as one would 'tea time' for relaxation, refreshment and communion with others."*

KIYOKO MORITA, *The Book of Incense*

In Japan, the highly ritualized Kodo incense appreciation ceremony is designed to cultivate aesthetic refinement while deepening spiritual awareness. In this context, incense is the muse of both enlightenment and artistic expression. The heart of Kodo is the practice of "listening to incense" — smelling with one's entire being.

As with the formal tea ceremony, it takes years to master the complexities of the "Way of Incense." There are specific rules regarding the subtleties of preparing the censer cup, pressing artistic designs into the white rice ash to correspond to the season and occasion, regulating the temperature of charcoal, blending the incense, and so on. An incense master must also draw upon a rich knowledge of poetry, classical literature, history, and natural science in order to fully comprehend and share the mysteries of incense. Gold-lacquered incense boxes inlaid with mother-of-pearl, exquisite Kodo burners, trays, and other ceremonial utensils can cost thousands of dollars.

The term *Kumiko* refers to the literary memory games of Kodo in which players must distinguish and identify different incenses by their perfume alone. David Oller, editor of *Incense Journal,* describes these games as being "aromatic journeys shared with a group of friends." He continues: "The true source of competition is to see which one among you is able to enjoy and cause the other participants to enjoy the journey the most."

There are hundreds of different Kumiko games that use various incenses and poetic procedures. These games are usually played with loose incense, such as aloeswood and sandalwood chips, using a Kodo-style censer cup filled with rice ash, charcoal, and a postage-stamp-sized mica plate to heat the slivers of precious incense. The following beginner-level games were suggested by Mark Ambrose of Scents of Earth.

### INTRODUCTORY GAME

#### Step One

The master of ceremonies prepares the incense censer and places three or four varieties of aloeswood in individual origami envelopes.

#### Step Two

Guests sit in a circle and pass each smoldering wood around for every person to experience. On the first pass, the host names each wood, giving it an evocative title like "Hidden Forest," "Autumn Wind," or "Snow on a Lonely Peak," and the guests try to associate the name with the scent. A designated record keeper writes down the name given to each wood on the inside of the origami envelopes in the order in which the varieties are passed.

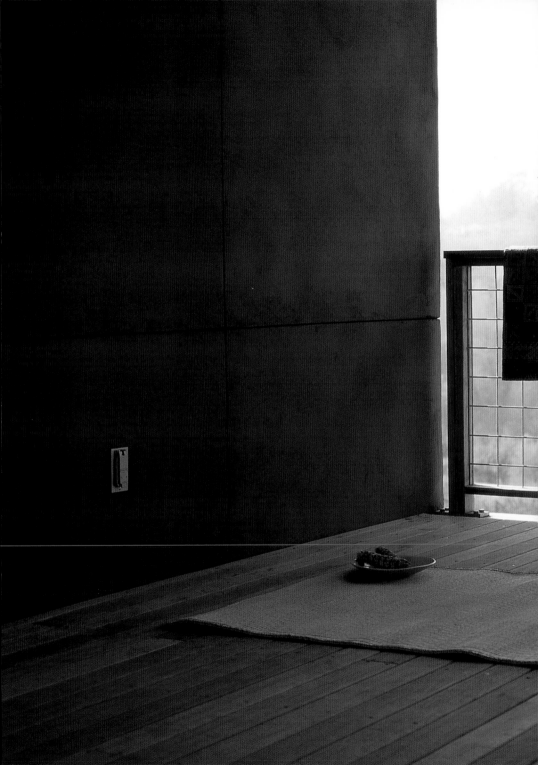

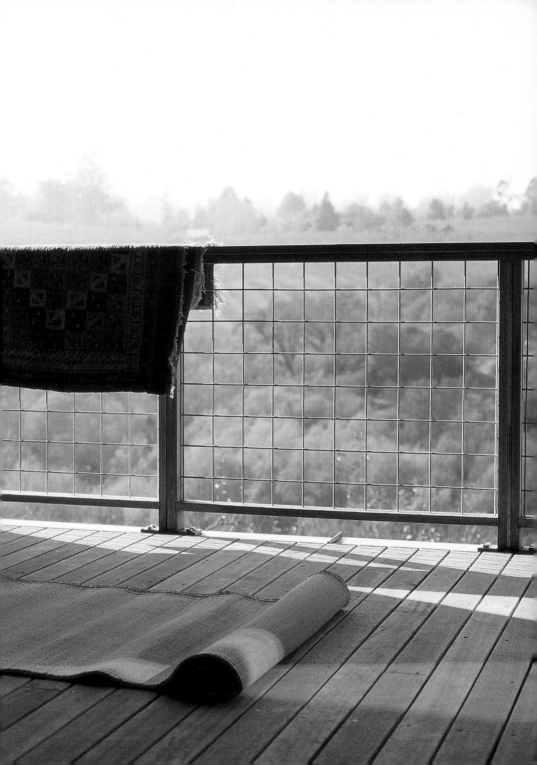

### Step Three

After each wood had been named and passed, the envelopes are then shuffled, and each wood is passed again, this time without a name. The guests then try to recall the name associated with the aroma and record it on their own beautiful slips of paper.

### Step Four

At the end of the game, the host opens each envelope and reads the names in the order in which the woods were initially passed. Each guest then discovers how well they associated the names with the fragrances.

## GAME OF THREE

### Step One

The master of ceremonies prepares the censer.

### Step Two

One at a time, three smoldering woods are passed around the circle.

### Step Three

The guests try to determine whether all three are different or two or more are the same.

## Poem in Four Scents

*Step One*

The master of ceremonies prepares the censer.

*Step Two*

One at a time, four smoldering woods are passed around the circle.

*Step Three*

When the first incense has been passed, the first guest writes a line of poetry inspired by the experience of "listening" to the fragrance. The next guest adds another line, the next guest adds a third, and so on, until all of the woods have been passed and a single poem has been created. Alternatively, participants can individually compose their own poems by writing down a line inspired by each incense, and then reading their four-line poems to one another.

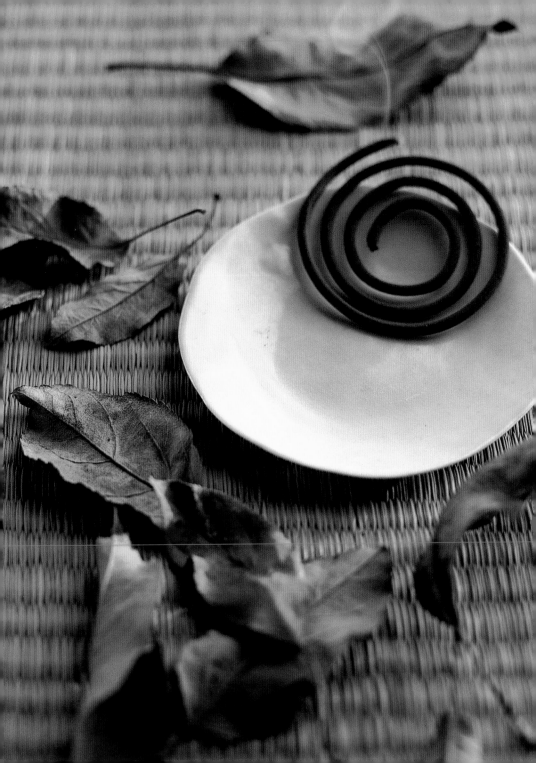

# 5 | Marking Time: Incense and Rites of Passage

Collectively, we remember certain kinds

of rites that our ancestors performed,

which, if resurrected in accordance with

our own aesthetics and circumstances,

add beauty to our lives

and bring us closer together.

ALFRED SAVINELLI, *PLANTS OF POWER*

## Marking Time: Incense and Rites of Passage

The belief that incense heightens awareness of the moment, summons the attention of deities, and provides inspirational comfort makes incense a natural component of rites of passage in many civilizations. Smoldering herbs and resins have been used to mark every stage of life.

What could be better than welcoming a baby to a world sweet with incense? Moroccans burn aloeswood on the day they name a child, and Sufis burn it to initiate a baby's soul into the depths of mysteries. North African mothers fumigate newborn babies' blankets with incense as protection against evil spirits. On the morning of the third day of a Chinese baby's life, the child is given his or her first bath. An offering of incense burns as the baby is bathed in warm water that has been boiled with locust branches; the child wears a silver or gold padlock around his or her neck, symbolically locking him or her to this world. You can also use gentle incense to lull a baby to sleep or to soothe a cranky toddler.

Arabic nomads shower brides-to-be with frankincense and saffron before their weddings, believing that these fragrances enhance fertility. In India, Hindu brides and grooms are enveloped by the smells of sandalwood and jasmine as they make their vows. Incense is a beautiful

element in any wedding celebration. A scented ambience creates a sense of ritual. The smoke of two incense sticks rising and mingling in the air can also reflect the couple's intention to live their lives as one.

Incense smoke is often present at seasonal rites of renewal. For instance, during Tet, the Vietnamese New Year, home altars burn with sandalwood and narcissus incense sticks. This elaborate three-day holiday is a time to give thanks and to ask for blessings. Families clean their homes and decorate them with chrysanthemums and peach blossoms. What happens during these days is thought to be an omen of the year to come, so everyone goes to great lengths to maintain a happy disposition, hoping that their dreams of happiness will come true as a result. During Tet, the first visitor to a home is considered very important; if the visitor is rich, then the family will have good fortune that year. Guests end their visit with a farewell wish for the family, such as, "I wish that money will flow into your house like water, and out like a turtle."

In China, the Kitchen God, Tsao Wang, is believed to offer protection from fire and all manner of culinary disasters, and to be the overseer of a household's moral conduct. Many Chinese families pay homage to him by placing a shrine on their kitchen wall or above the stove. He is usually depicted as an ornately costumed nobleman standing beside a handsome steed. People pray to the Kitchen God with offerings of incense, candles, and sweets, believing that during Chinese Lunar New Year the Kitchen God travels to heaven to report to the Jade Emperor on the moral behavior of each family member during the past year. He is thought to ride up to heaven on the whorl of smoke created by people burning his portrait. In this burning ritual, incense is used to represent the provisions he will need on the journey, and hay is sometimes spread out to represent feed for his horse. Before setting the Kitchen God's image on fire, people smear his lips with honey, hoping that doing so will make him say only sweet things about them. Those who have been especially bad sometimes give him a great deal of honey, attempting to seal his lips shut so he can't say anything at all!

*Naw Ruz,* literally "New Day," marks the new year for people of all faiths in Iran and Afghanistan. It begins on the vernal equinox, which usually happens on March 21. The centerpiece of the holiday is a ceremonial table laid with seven dishes that all begin with the Persian letter *S.* The number seven has been considered sacred in Persia since ancient times, and the seven dishes stand for the seven angelic heralds of life: rebirth, health, happiness, prosperity, joy, patience, and beauty.

The ceremonial dishes include:

*sabzeh* (bright green wheat or lentil sprouts), which represents rebirth and prosperity

*samanu* (a sweet, creamy pudding made from wheat sprouts), which symbolizes fertility and growth

*seeb* (apple), which symbolizes health and beauty

*senjed* (the sweet, dry fruit of the lotus tree), which represents shelter, love, and security

*seer* (garlic), which symbolizes peace

*Sumac berries,* which are the color of sunrise and represent good conquering evil

*serkeh* (vinegar), which represents patience

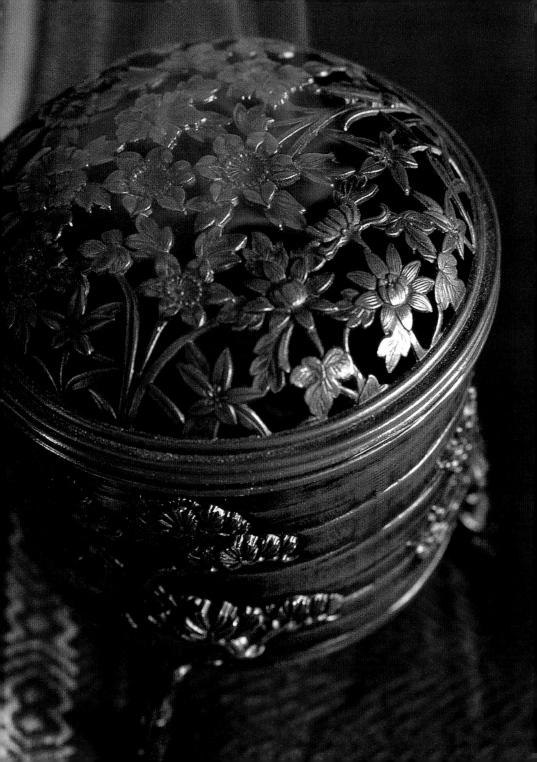

In addition to these foods, the table is decorated with a variety of other symbolic items, among them a mirror, a bowl with live goldfish, painted eggs, candles, and incense. The fragrance of the incense is thought to help celebrants meditate and pray.

Since ancient times, when the Egyptians treated their mummies with the smoke of herbs to send them into the next life, incense and death have gone hand in hand. Many cultures have a long history of incorporating incense into their cremation ceremonies. Incense masks the stench of a burning body and accompanies the soul on its journey to the next realm. The ancient Romans burned lavender on their funeral pyres. The Greeks burned iris root so that Iris, goddess of the rainbow and messenger of the gods, would escort the dead person's spirit along the rainbow into the "Land of Everlasting Peace."

Hindu families in Bali and India add precious sandalwood to their cremation pyres. Buddhists burn incense in the presence of a corpse to shield it and the newly parted soul from malevolent demons. During Catholic funeral masses, priests incense the corpse or cremated remains with frankincense as a sign of reverence for the body that was once the temple of God.

Families in Mexico, Vietnam, China, Taiwan, and many other countries bring offerings of incense and flowers to cemeteries to pay respect to their deceased ancestors and friends. The incense is thought to open channels of communication with the dead, carrying prayers and fond memories, along with the latest family gossip for the departed to enjoy.

## Create a Memorial Altar

Create a memorial shrine in your home to help you remember your deceased loved ones. Memorial altars usually include a portrait of the honoree and candles, in addition to incense. You might also consider decorating yours with items that evoke the memory of your beloved — his or her baseball cap, a torn ticket stub from a movie you attended together, a shell from his or her favorite beach. You can burn incense on the altar to commune with your loved one's spirit every day or just to mark special occasions like birthdays, anniversaries, and holidays. In Mexico and Vietnam, people sometimes prepare the foods that the dead most enjoyed in life and place these dishes as an offering on the altar. Lured back to earth by the festive incense and food, the spirits are said to rejoice in the delicious aromas.

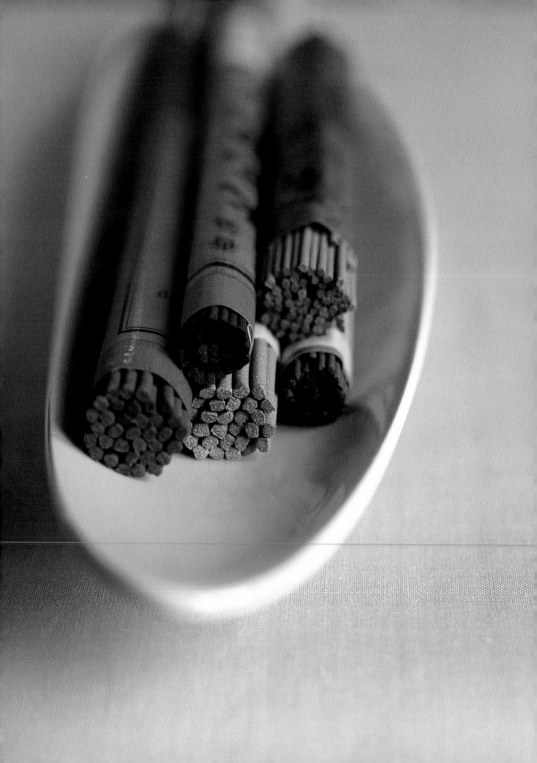

## Incense Resources

**Adventure Arabia**
2 Bullfinch Close
Creekmoor, Poole
Dorset BH17 7UP
United Kingdom
44/120-246-2021
www.adventurearabia.com

**Asakichi Incense**
Japan Center
1730 Geary Blvd.
Suite 206A
San Francisco, CA 94115
415/921-8292

**Baieido Co., Ltd.**
1-1-4 Kurumano-cho
Higashi
Sakai City, Osaka
590-0943
Japan
0722/29-4545
www.baieido.co.jp/english

**Enfleurage**
321 Bleecker Street
New York, NY 10014
888/387-0300
www.enfleurage.com

**The Kodo Store**
(online only)
www.kodostore.com

**Mere Cie**
1100 Soscol Ferry
   Road, #3
Napa, CA 94558
800/832-4544
www.merecie.com

**Mother's Hearth**
3443 East 11th Street
Tulsa, OK 74112
918/835-3290
www.makeincense.com

**Native Scents, Inc.**
P.O. Box 5639
Taos, NM 87571
800/645-3471
www.nativescents.com

**NipponKodo, Inc.**
2771 Plaza Del Amo,
   Suite 806
Torrance, CA 90503
888/775-5487
www.nipponkodo.com

**PaulaWalla Imports**
180 Rainbow Road
Windsor, CT 06095
860/490-4258
www.paulawalla.com

**Prasad Gifts, Inc.**
502 South Fourth Street
Fairfield, IA 52556
800/772-7231
www.prasadgifts.com

**Scents of Earth**
P.O. Box 859
Sun City, CA 92586
800/323-8159
www.scents-of-earth.com

**Sensia, Inc./Good Scents**
327 Carpenters Lane
Cape May, NJ 08204
800/777-8027
www.sensia.com

**Shoyeido**
1700 38th Street
Boulder, CO 80301
800/786-5476
www.shoyeido.com

## Incense Aromatherapy Chart

| Ingredient | Scent | Mood |
| --- | --- | --- |
| Aloeswood | Woody | Calming, spiritual |
| Ambrette Seeds | Musk | Romantic, balancing |
| Basil | Spicy | Clarity of thought |
| Benzoin | Balsamic | Comforting |
| Borneo Camphor | Woody | Refreshing |
| Cardamom | Spicy | Romantic |
| Cedarwood | Woody | Comforting |
| Cinnamon | Spicy | Emotionally uplifting, restorative |
| Citronella | Citrus | Soothing |
| Clary Sage | Herbal | Confidence, peace |
| Clove | Spicy | Energizing |
| Dragon's Blood | Herbal | Purifying |
| Frankincense | Resinous | Spiritual |
| Gardenia | Floral | Uplifting |
| Ginger | Spicy | Revitalizing |
| Honeysuckle | Floral | Cheerful, romantic |
| Jasmine | Floral | Balancing |
| Juniper | Spicy | Restorative |
| Lavender | Herbal | Calming |

| Ingredient | Scent | Mood |
| --- | --- | --- |
| Lemongrass | Citrus | Energizing |
| Musk Thistle Flowers | Musk | Romantic |
| Myrrh | Resinous | Calming, restorative |
| Myrtle | Spicy | Forgiveness, emotional healing |
| Oakmoss | Earthy | Cleansing |
| Orange Blossom | Floral | Balancing, cheerful |
| Patchouli | Earthy | Joy |
| Peru balsam | Balsamic | Comforting |
| Pine | Woody | Refreshing, restorative |
| Rose | Floral | Well-being |
| Rosemary | Herbal | Clarity |
| Sandalwood | Woody | Uplifting, sensual |
| Spikenard Root | Musk | Relaxing |
| Storax | Balsamic | May relieve sleeplessness |
| Sweet Grass | Herbal | Cleansing |
| Tolu balsam | Balsamic | Comforting |
| Vetiver | Earthy | Calming, balancing |
| White Lotus | Floral | Revitalizing |
| Ylang-Ylang | Floral | Soothing, calming |

# Bibliography

ACKERMAN, DIANE. *A Natural History of the Senses.* New York: Vintage, 1990.

AFTEL, MANDY. *Essence and Alchemy: A Book of Perfume.* New York: North Point Press, 2001.

BABCOCK, PHILIP G. *Webster's Third New International Dictionary of the English Language.* Springfield, Mass.: Merriam-Webster, Inc., 1986.

BEDINI, SILVIO A. *The Scent of Time: A Study of the Use of Fire and Incense for Time Measurement in Oriental Countries.* Transactions of the American Philosophical Society, n.s., 53, pt. 5. Philadelphia, 1963.

BREE, WITCH. *Witch's Brew: Good Spells for Love.* San Francisco: Chronicle Books LLC, 2001.

CRUDEN, LOREN. *Medicine Grove: A Shamanic Herbal.* Rochester, Vt.: Destiny Books, 1997.

FELLNER, TARA. *Aromatherapy for Lovers: Essential Recipes for Romance.* Boston: Journey Editions, 1995.

FETTNER, ANNE TUCKER. *Potpourri, Incense and Other Fragrant Concoctions.* New York: Workman Publishing Company, 1977.

FISCHER-RIZZI, SUSANNE. *The Complete Incense Book.* New York: Sterling Publishing Co., Inc., 1998.

FRONTY, LAURA. *The Scented Home: Natural Recipes in the French Tradition.* New York: Universe Publishing, 2002.

GROOM, NIGEL. *Frankincense and Myrrh.* Essex, England: Longman Group Limited, 1981.

HIRSCH, ALAN R. *Scentsational Sex.* Boston: Element, 1998.

LAKE, MAX. *Scents and Sexuality.* London: Futura, 1991.

LAWLESS, JULIA. *Aromatherapy and the Mind.* London: Thorsons, 1994.

LINN, DENISE. *Space Clearing: How to Purify and Create Harmony in Your Home.* Lincolnwood, Ill.: Contemporary Books, 2000.

MORITA, KIYOKO. *The Book of Incense: Enjoying the Traditional Art of Japanese Scents.* New York: Kodansha International, Ltd., 1992.

MORRIS, EDWIN T. *Fragrance: The Story of Perfume from Cleopatra to Chanel.* New York: Charles Scribner's Sons, 1984.

OLLER, DAVID. *The Incense Journal.* Online magazine dedicated to the art and practice of incense appreciation and blending: www.oller.net/incense/journal.htm

PYBUS, DAVID. *Kodo: The Way of Incense.* Boston: Tuttle Publishing, 2001.

ROSEN, DIANA. *The Essence of Incense: Bringing Fragrance into the Home.* North Adams, Mass.: Storey Books, 2001.

SAVINELLI, ALFRED. *Plants of Power: Native American Ceremony and the Use of Sacred Plants.* Summertown, Tenn.: Native Voices, 2002.

SHIKIBU, MURASAKI. *The Tale of Genji.* Translated by Edward G. Seidensticker. New York: Alfred A. Knopf, 1983.

SMITH, STEVEN R. *Wylundt's Book of Incense.* York Beach, Maine: Samuel Weiser, Inc., 1989.

STREEP, PEG. *Altars Made Easy: A Complete Guide to Creating Your Own Sacred Space.* New York: HarperCollins Publishers, 1997.

# Index

## Acknowledgments

Heartfelt thanks to editor Lisa Campbell for shepherding this project to fruition with great care and thoughtfulness, and to research assistant extraordinaire Megan Flautt, whose mania for all things incense was a source of constant delight. A writer couldn't ask for a more inspired design team: photographer Susie Cushner, photo stylist Sara Slavin, and designers Meg Coughlin and Vivien Sung each contributed their artistry to this project. Thanks as well to copy editor Karen O'Donnell Stein, in-house sachet expert Susan Coyle, Lisa Bach, Jan Hughes, Leslie Jonath, Doug Ogan, Nion McEvoy, Beth Steiner, and the rest of the swell gang at Chronicle Books.

For their generous assistance with both research information and sample materials, I'm tremendously grateful to Mark Ambrose of Scents of Earth; Dan Andrews of Mere Cie; Jeff Banach of Shoyeido; Trygve Harris of Enfleurage; Cindy Huf of Sensia, Inc.; David Oller of Esoterics LLC; Einar Olsen of Prasad Gifts, Inc.; Paula Pierce of PaulaWalla Imports; Alfred Savinelli of Native Scents, Inc.; and Roland Torikian of Centro Maya. For their steadfast support on the home front, I'm grateful as ever to Dave and Annalena Barrett and Leigh Hyams (my sweet myrrh, my cinnamon, and my copal) and to my wise and kind agent Amy Rennert. Finally, I get by with a lot of help from my girlfriends: *besitos* to Anne Burt, Susan Davis, and Robin Tremblay-McGaw. —GINA HYAMS

Making photographs to illustrate a book requires a unique and seasoned group of people. They must possess balance, passion, and a feel for effortless creation by focusing attention on the project and accomplishing a complete thought in a limited timeframe. I extend honor and gratitude to my dear friend Sara Slavin for agreeing to take this project on and bringing the energy and creativity that only she can, along with her friends and resources that were gracious in their contributions: Barbara Vick for allowing us to shoot in her extraordinary home; Steven and Del from Dandelion in San Francisco; The Gardener in Berkeley; Asakichi Incense and Shige Kimonos in the Japan Center, San Francisco. I also wish to thank my assistant and friend, Meg Matyia, and MD for generously opening her home to us in her absence. A special thanks to Sara's husband, Mark Steisel, for putting up with the invasion, letting me light the Chanukah candles and having the best nature! THANK YOU ALL. — SUSIE CUSHNER